Look Younger Forever

"The Secrets to Staying Young and Radiant"

Dr. Frank Jameson

Table Of Contents

Introduction

Aging Process of Humans

Nutrition and diet for optimal skin, hair, and overall health

Exercise and physical activity for maintaining a youthful physique

Skincare routine and products for preventing and reversing signs of aging

Makeup techniques for accentuating natural beauty and minimizing the appearance of aging

Mindfulness and stress management for promoting overall well-being

Alternative treatments such as acupuncture, hormone therapy, and anti-aging supplements

The role of genetics in aging and strategies for maximizing your potential

The role of genetics in aging is complex and multi-faceted.

Conclusion and final tips for maintaining a youthful, radiant appearance

Introduction

Introduction to the concept of "Look Younger Forever" and the importance of maintaining a youthful appearance

Look younger Forever " is a phrase that refers to the idea of remaining youthful and vibrant indefinitely. It is often associated with physical appearance, and people may strive to maintain a youthful appearance through various means such as exercise, diet, skincare, and cosmetics. There is also a cultural significance attached to the phrase, with many people believing that looking youthful is desirable and can be linked to success, attractiveness, and vitality. Some people may also associate the concept of "forever young" with a desire for longevity and a fear of aging.

The concept of "Looking Younger Forever" is often associated with the desire to maintain a youthful appearance, as well as a desire for longevity and good health. While it is not possible to truly remain forever young, there are a number of ways that people can try to slow down the aging process and improve their health and well-being.

Some of the most popular ways to try to stay "forever young" include:

Eating a healthy diet: A diet rich in fruits, vegetables, and whole grains can help to reduce the risk of age-related diseases and promote overall health.

Exercise: Regular physical activity can help to keep the body in good shape and reduce the risk of age-related diseases.

Managing stress: Chronic stress has been linked to an increased risk of age-related diseases, so finding ways to manage stress is important.

Getting enough sleep: Sleep plays an important role in overall health, and getting enough restful sleep can help to reduce the risk of age-related diseases.

Avoiding smoking and excessive alcohol consumption: Both smoking and excessive alcohol consumption have been linked to an increased risk of age-related diseases.

Proper skincare and use of cosmetics: Proper skincare and use of cosmetics can help to keep the skin looking youthful, but it's important to use products that are safe and appropriate for your skin type.

It's important to note that while these practices may help to slow down the aging process, they cannot truly stop it, and that the ultimate goal should be to age healthily and gracefully.

Maintaining a youthful appearance can be important for a variety of reasons. Some people may want to look young to feel more attractive or to boost their confidence. In some cultures, there is a societal expectation that people should look young, and those who do not may be stigmatized. Additionally, people may believe that looking young is associated with success and vitality.

In some industries, such as entertainment or modeling, there may be pressure to maintain a youthful appearance in order to remain competitive. Some people may also feel that looking young can help them to be taken more seriously in the workplace.

However, it's important to note that there is also a negative side to the emphasis on youth and appearance. Society can often discriminate against older people, and this can be harmful. People should also be aware that there are no scientific proof that external appearance can affect internal health, and that the focus on youth can be harmful for mental health and self-esteem.

Aging Process of Humans

The aging process is a complex biological process that occurs over time. It is characterized by a gradual decline in the body's ability to function properly, leading to an increased risk of disease and death.

There are several factors that contribute to the aging process. One of the most significant is genetics. Our genes play a large role in determining how our bodies age, and inherited genetic variations can make some people more susceptible to age-related diseases.

Another major factor that contributes to the aging process is *oxidative stress*, which is caused by an imbalance between the production of reactive oxygen species and the body's ability to neutralize them. This can lead to cellular damage, which over time can contribute to the development of age-related diseases.

Aging is also influenced by lifestyle choices and environmental factors. Poor diet, lack of physical activity, exposure to toxins, chronic stress and smoking are some of the lifestyle factors that can contribute to the aging process.

Finally, telomeres, the protective caps at the end of chromosomes, shorten as we age. This leads to a decline in cell division and ultimately contributes to aging.

It's important to note that aging is a natural process and cannot be stopped, but a healthy lifestyle and environmental factors can help to slow down the aging process and improve quality of life in old age.

There are several other factors that contribute to the aging process, including:

Inflammation: Chronic inflammation has been linked to several age-related diseases, including heart disease, diabetes, and cancer.

Hormones: Hormones play a critical role in the aging process. As we age, our hormone levels decline, which can lead to a variety of age-related changes in the body.

Metabolism: As we age, our metabolism slows down, which can lead to weight gain and an increased risk of age-related diseases.

Microorganisms: The presence of certain microorganisms in the body has been linked to the aging process. For example,

the accumulation of certain types of
bacteria in the gut has been associated
with an increased risk of age-related
diseases.

Sleep: Poor sleep quality and a lack of
sleep have been linked to an increased risk
of age-related diseases.

Social interactions: Studies have shown
that social isolation and loneliness can
contribute to the aging process.

Mental health: Stress, depression, and
anxiety have been linked to an increased
risk of age-related diseases and a shorter
lifespan.

It's important to note that while aging is a
complex process influenced by multiple
factors, genetics plays a major role in the

rate at which we age. Also, the factors
mentioned above can interact and have a
synergistic effect on aging.

Nutrition and diet for optimal skin, hair, and overall health

Nutrition and diet play a crucial role in maintaining optimal skin, hair, and overall health. A diet that is rich in vitamins, minerals, and antioxidants can help to nourish the skin and hair, while also supporting overall health and wellness.

Here are some key nutrients that are important for maintaining healthy skin, hair, and overall health:

Vitamin C: Vitamin C is essential for the production of collagen, which is a protein that helps to keep the skin firm and elastic. It can also help to protect the skin from damage caused by the sun and pollution. Foods that are high in vitamin C include oranges, strawberries, kiwi, bell peppers, and spinach.

Vitamin E: Vitamin E is an antioxidant that helps to protect the skin from damage caused by free radicals. It also helps to keep the skin moisturized and can improve the appearance of fine lines and wrinkles. Foods that are high in vitamin E include almonds, sunflower seeds, and avocado.

Vitamin A: Vitamin A is important for the growth and repair of skin cells. It can also help to reduce the appearance of fine lines and wrinkles. Foods that are high in vitamin A include carrots, sweet potatoes, and leafy greens.

Omega-3 fatty acids: Omega-3 fatty acids are essential for maintaining healthy skin, hair, and nails. They can also help to reduce inflammation and improve overall health. Foods that are high in omega-3 fatty acids include fatty fish such as salmon, flaxseeds, and chia seeds.

Zinc: Zinc is important for maintaining healthy skin, hair, and nails. It also helps to support the immune system and can improve overall health. Foods that are high in zinc include oysters, beef, and pumpkin seeds.

Protein: Protein is essential for the growth and repair of skin, hair, and nails. Foods that are high in protein include fish, chicken, eggs, and legumes.

It's important to keep in mind that a balanced diet that includes a variety of nutrient-dense foods is key for optimal skin, hair, and overall health, and that supplements should be taken under professional guidance.

In addition to the key nutrients mentioned above, there are several other important factors to consider when it comes to nutrition and diet for optimal skin, hair, and overall health.

Hydration: Drinking enough water is essential for maintaining healthy skin, hair, and nails. It helps to keep the skin hydrated and can help to flush out toxins from the body. Aim to drink at least 8-10 glasses of water per day.

Fiber: Eating a diet that is high in fiber can help to promote healthy digestion and regular bowel movements. This can help to keep the skin looking clear and reduce the risk of acne.

Antioxidants: Antioxidants help to protect the skin from damage caused by free radicals. Eating a diet that is rich in antioxidants can help to reduce the risk of age-related diseases and improve overall health. Berries, dark leafy greens, and dark chocolate are all high in antioxidants.

Probiotics: Probiotics are beneficial bacteria that live in the gut. Consuming probiotics through fermented foods such as yogurt, kefir, and sauerkraut can help to promote a healthy gut microbiome, which in turn is essential for overall health and wellbeing.

Avoiding processed foods and added sugars: Processed foods and added sugars can contribute to inflammation in the body, which can lead to skin problems and other health issues. To keep skin and overall health optimal, it's best to avoid processed foods and added sugars as much as possible and opt for whole, nutrient-dense foods instead.

It's important to remember that everyone's nutritional needs are different, and that it's best to work with a healthcare professional or a registered dietitian to create a personalized plan that meets your specific needs.
(Note: Check out my book on Amazon store" Diets that makes you look younger")

Exercise and physical activity for maintaining a youthful physique

Exercise and physical activity are essential for maintaining a youthful physique. Regular exercise can help to improve muscle tone, increase strength, reduce body fat, and improve overall cardiovascular health. A combination of cardio, strength training, and stretching is ideal for maintaining a youthful physique.

Cardio exercises such as running,cycling, and swimming can help to improve cardiovascular fitness, while strength training exercises such as weightlifting, resistance band training, and bodyweight exercises can help to build and maintain muscle mass. Stretching is also important for maintaining flexibility and preventing injury. It is also important to maintain a healthy diet, stay well-hydrated, and get enough sleep to support overall health and fitness.

It's also important to vary your exercise routine to avoid boredom and to target different muscle groups. This can include activities such as yoga, Pilates, or dance classes. Additionally, incorporating balance and coordination exercises can help to improve overall stability and reduce the risk of falls as we age.

To maintain a youthful physique, it is recommended to engage in at least 30 minutes of moderate-intensity physical activity most days of the week, and to include both cardio and strength training exercises in your routine. It's also important to stay consistent with your exercise routine and to make it a part of your daily or weekly routine. Remember that physical activity is not only beneficial for maintaining a youthful physique, but also for overall health and well-being.

Here are some examples of exercises that can help you maintain a youthful physique:

Cardio: Running, cycling, swimming, and dancing are all great cardio exercises that can improve cardiovascular fitness and help to burn calories.

Strength Training: Weightlifting, resistance band training, and bodyweight exercises (such as push-ups and squats) are great for building and maintaining muscle mass.

Yoga: Yoga is a great exercise for improving flexibility and balance, and it can also help to reduce stress and improve overall well-being.

Pilates: Pilates is a form of exercise that focuses on core strength, balance, and flexibility, which can help to tone and sculpt the body.

High-intensity interval training (HIIT): This type of training typically involves short bursts of intense activity followed by brief periods of recovery. It can be effective at burning calories and improving cardiovascular fitness.

Resistance training: This type of training can increase muscle mass, improve bone density and overall strength, which will make you look and feel younger.

Flexibility exercises: Stretching exercises can help to improve overall flexibility and reduce the risk of injury.

It is important to note that everyone has different fitness levels and physical capabilities, so it's important to consult with a doctor or professional trainer before starting a new exercise program. Also, it's essential to listen to your body and not to overdo it, gradually increase the intensity and duration of your exercise routine over time.

Skincare routine and products for preventing and reversing signs of aging

A skincare routine that includes using the right products can help to prevent and even reverse the signs of aging. Here are some key steps and products to consider:

Cleansing: It is important to cleanse the skin twice a day to remove dirt, oil, and makeup. A gentle, non-foaming cleanser is recommended.

Exfoliating: Exfoliating helps to remove dead skin cells, which can improve the appearance of fine lines and wrinkles. A gentle, chemical exfoliant such as alpha-hydroxy acids (AHAs) or beta-hydroxy acids (BHAs) can be used 1-2 times a week.

Moisturizing: Keeping the skin hydrated is important for preventing and reversing signs of aging. A lightweight, water-based moisturizer can be used during the day, and a thicker, oil-based moisturizer can be used at night.

Sunscreen: Sun exposure can accelerate the aging process, so it is important to use a sunscreen with at least SPF 30 every day.

Eye cream: The skin around the eyes is thin and delicate, so a separate eye cream can help to hydrate and reduce the appearance of fine lines and wrinkles.

Retinoids: Retinoids are derived from Vitamin A and can help to improve the appearance of fine lines, wrinkles, and uneven skin tone. They can be very effective, but they can be irritating to the skin, so it is best to start with a low-strength formulation and use them at night.

Antioxidants: Antioxidants such as Vitamin C and E can help to protect the skin from free radical damage and can also help to improve the appearance of fine lines and wrinkles.

Collagen Boosters: Collagen is a protein that gives skin its structure, elasticity and firmness. As we age, collagen production decreases, leading to wrinkles and sagging. There are some products like retinoids and Vitamin C that have been shown to boost collagen production, but there are also dietary supplements like marine collagen that can help.

It's important to note that everyone's skin is different, so it's important to consult with a dermatologist or skincare professional to find the best skincare routine and products for your individual needs.

In addition to the skincare routine and products mentioned earlier, here are a few more notes to keep in mind when it comes to preventing and reversing the signs of aging:

Be consistent: A consistent skincare routine is key to seeing results. It's important to stick to a regular routine and not to skip steps or products.

Use gentle products: Avoid using harsh or abrasive products on the skin, as they can cause irritation and inflammation, which can accelerate the aging process.

Avoid smoking and excessive alcohol consumption: Both smoking and excessive alcohol consumption can contribute to the aging of the skin, so it's best to avoid or limit these habits as much as possible.

Get enough sleep: Adequate sleep is essential for overall health and well-being, and it can also help to improve the appearance of the skin.

Eat a healthy diet: Eating a diet rich in fruits, vegetables, and healthy fats can help to nourish the skin from within and support skin health.

Stay hydrated: Drinking plenty of water can help to keep the skin hydrated and plump, which can help to reduce the appearance of fine lines and wrinkles.

Be mindful of your environment: Being aware of your environment and taking steps to protect your skin from pollution and UV rays can help to prevent damage and slow the aging process.

Consider professional treatments: Professional treatments such as chemical peels, microdermabrasion, and laser resurfacing can be effective at improving the appearance of fine lines and wrinkles, but they should be done under the supervision of a skincare professional.

Monitor your skincare products: Keep an eye on the expiration date of the skincare products you're using, as they can lose their effectiveness over time. Also, pay attention to how your skin reacts to certain products and adjust accordingly.

It's also important to remember that aging is a natural process, and it is impossible to completely stop the aging process, but with the right skincare routine and healthy lifestyle choices, you can help to prevent and reverse the signs of aging.

Makeup techniques for accentuating natural beauty and minimizing the appearance of aging

Makeup can be used to accentuate natural beauty and minimize the appearance of aging. Here are a few makeup techniques to consider:

Use a lightweight, oil-free foundation: A lightweight, oil-free foundation can help to even out skin tone and create a natural-looking base without clogging pores or settling into fine lines and wrinkles.

Conceal dark circles and age spots: Concealer can be used to brighten up dark circles and age spots, which can make the skin look more youthful.

Highlight and contour: Highlighting and contouring can be used to create the illusion of a more youthful face by adding depth and dimension to the skin. By highlighting the high points of the face and contouring the hollows, you can create a more youthful, lifted appearance.

Apply blush: A pop of blush on the apples of the cheeks can help to add color and life to the face, which can make the skin look more youthful.

Use a lip plumper: A lip plumper can be used to add fullness to the lips, which can make the face look more youthful.

Apply eyeliner: Applying eyeliner can help to define the eyes and make them look more youthful.

Use mascara: A coat of mascara can help to open up the eyes and make them look more youthful.

Use a powder: A powder can help to set your makeup and keep it in place all day, so your skin will look fresh and youthful.

Use a primer: A primer can help to create a smooth base for your makeup, which can help to minimize the appearance of fine lines and wrinkles.

Use a setting spray: A setting spray can help to keep your makeup in place all day, which can help to minimize the appearance of aging.

Use a brow pencil: A brow pencil can be used to fill in and shape the brows, which can help to frame the face and make the eyes look more youthful.

Use a bronzer: A bronzer can be used to add warmth and dimension to the skin, which can make the face look more youthful.

Use a highlighter: A highlighter can be used to add a youthful glow to the skin, which can make the face look more youthful.

Use a lip gloss: A lip gloss can be used to add shine and fullness to the lips, which can make the face look more youthful.

Use a neutral eye shadow: A neutral eye shadow can be used to create a natural, youthful look that can be worn day or night.

Use a translucent powder: A translucent powder can be used to set your makeup and reduce shine, which can help to minimize the appearance of aging.

Use waterproof makeup: Waterproof makeup can help to keep your makeup in place and prevent smudging, which can help to minimize the appearance of aging.

It's important to remember that less is more when it comes to makeup and accentuating natural beauty. Use makeup to enhance your natural features and not to change them. Also, be mindful of the quality of the makeup products you use and ensure they are non-comedogenic and hypoallergenic.

Be mindful of the colors you use: Using colors that complement your skin tone can help to enhance your natural beauty and minimize the appearance of aging.

It's important to remember that everyone's skin is different, so it's best to experiment with different makeup techniques and products to find what works best for you. And, as with skincare, it's always best to work with a professional makeup artist to get personalized recommendations.

Mindfulness and stress management for promoting overall well-being

Mindfulness and stress management are important for promoting overall well-being. Here are a few techniques to consider:

Practice mindfulness: Mindfulness is the practice of being present in the moment and paying attention to your thoughts, feelings, and bodily sensations. Mindfulness can help to reduce stress, improve focus and concentration, and promote overall well-being.

Meditate: Meditation is a form of mindfulness that involves sitting in a comfortable position and focusing on your breath or a mantra. Meditation can help to reduce stress and anxiety, improve focus and concentration, and promote overall well-being.

Practice yoga: Yoga is a form of exercise that combines movement, breathing, and meditation. Yoga can help to reduce stress, improve flexibility and balance, and promote overall well-being.

Get enough sleep: Adequate sleep is essential for overall well-being. Lack of sleep can contribute to stress, anxiety, and depression, and can also affect cognitive function, mood, and physical health.

*Taking breaks:*Taking regular breaks throughout the day can help to reduce stress and improve focus and concentration.

Practice deep breathing: Deep breathing is a simple and effective way to reduce stress and promote relaxation.

Engage in regular exercise: Regular physical activity can help to reduce stress and improve overall well-being.

Practice gratitude: Practicing gratitude can help to shift your focus away from negative thoughts and towards positive aspects of your life.

Connect with others: Connecting with friends, family, or a support group can help to reduce stress and promote overall well-being.

It's important to remember that everyone's stress response is different, so it's best to experiment with different techniques and find what works best for you.

Mindfulness, stress management, and overall well-being are interrelated, so it's important to integrate all these in your daily routine.

Alternative treatments such as acupuncture, hormone therapy, and anti-aging supplements

Acupuncture, hormone therapy, and anti-aging supplements are alternative treatments that are often used to promote overall well-being and potentially reverse the signs of aging.

Acupuncture: Acupuncture is a traditional Chinese medicine technique that involves the insertion of thin needles into specific points on the body to promote healing and well-being. It's believed to help balance the flow of energy, called Qi, in the body and can be used to relieve pain, reduce stress and anxiety and improve overall well-being.

Hormone therapy: Hormone therapy is a treatment that involves the replacement or manipulation of hormones in the body. As we age, hormone levels decline, which can lead to a variety of symptoms such as fatigue, weight gain and decreased libido. Hormone therapy aims to restore these levels to a more youthful state. It is important to note that hormone therapy should only be done under the supervision of a qualified healthcare professional.

Anti-aging supplements: Anti-aging supplements are a popular alternative treatment that is designed to promote overall well-being and potentially reverse the signs of aging. These supplements usually contain a variety of vitamins, minerals, and other nutrients that are believed to be beneficial for aging skin and overall health. Some examples include omega-3 fatty acids, antioxidants, and collagen. It's important to note that supplements should be taken under the supervision of a healthcare professional and to be aware of the possible side effects.

It's important to note that alternative treatments are not always scientifically proven and may not be suitable for everyone. It is always recommended to talk with a healthcare professional before starting any alternative treatment to ensure that it is safe and appropriate for you.

The role of genetics in aging and strategies for maximizing your potential

The role of genetics in aging is complex and multi-faceted. Research has shown that genetics can play a significant role in determining how quickly we age and our risk for certain age-related diseases. However, it is important to note that genetics is not the only factor that determines how we age. Lifestyle choices and environmental factors also play a significant role.

There are certain genetic variations that are associated with a longer lifespan, such as those related to the sirtuin genes, which are known to regulate the aging process. However, having these variations does not guarantee a longer lifespan, and other factors such as diet and exercise can also affect the expression of these genes.

Despite the role of genetics in aging, there are still strategies that can be used to maximize one's potential and promote overall well-being. These include:

Eating a healthy diet: A diet that is rich in fruits, vegetables, lean protein, and whole grains can help to promote overall health and potentially slow the aging process.

Regular physical activity: Regular physical activity can help to improve cardiovascular health, reduce the risk of certain age-related diseases, and promote overall well-being.

Getting enough sleep: Getting enough sleep is essential for maintaining overall health, and lack of sleep has been linked to a number of age-related diseases.

Managing stress: Chronic stress can have a negative impact on overall health, and it's important to find effective ways to manage stress in order to promote overall well-being.

Not smoking: Smoking is a major risk factor for many age-related diseases, and quitting smoking can have a significant impact on overall health.

Regular medical check-ups: Regular medical check-ups can help to identify and address any potential health problems early on.

It is also worth noting that some genetic test can be done to identify the genetic variations related to aging and disease risks. These test can give you some information about your risk but it's important to consider that test results are not the only factor in determining one's health outcomes. Your lifestyle and environmental factors can have a big impact on your health outcomes and test results should be used as a guide and not a definite answer.

In addition to the strategies mentioned above, there are other ways to potentially maximize one's potential and promote overall well-being despite the role of genetics in aging.

Personalized medicine: With advances in genetic testing and personalized medicine, it is now possible to identify specific genetic variations that may increase one's risk for certain age-related diseases. This information can then be used to tailor treatment and prevention strategies to an individual's specific needs.

Telomere testing: Telomeres are the protective caps on the ends of chromosomes that shorten as we age, and telomere length has been linked to aging and age-related diseases. Telomere testing can help to identify individuals who may be at an increased risk for certain age-related diseases and can be used to tailor prevention and treatment strategies.

Epigenetics: Epigenetics refers to the study of how environmental factors can affect the expression of genes. By understanding how environmental factors such as diet and exercise can affect gene expression, it may be possible to find ways to slow the aging process and reduce the risk of certain age-related diseases.

Stem cell therapy: Stem cell therapy is an experimental treatment that involves the use of stem cells to repair or replace damaged cells in the body. Stem cells have the ability to divide and differentiate into different cell types, which makes them a promising treatment option for age-related diseases.

It is important to note that while these strategies may have potential benefits, they are still largely experimental and may not be suitable for everyone. It is always recommended to talk with a healthcare professional before starting any new treatment or therapy to ensure that it is safe and appropriate for you.

Conclusion and final tips for maintaining a youthful, radiant appearance

Maintaining a youthful, radiant appearance is a combination of several factors including genetics, lifestyle choices, and skincare routine. While genetics plays a role in determining how we age, there are still steps that can be taken to promote overall well-being and potentially slow the aging process.

Some final tips for maintaining a youthful, radiant appearance include:

Adopting a healthy lifestyle: Eating a healthy diet, getting regular exercise, getting enough sleep, and managing stress are all important for maintaining overall health and potentially slowing the aging process.

Using skincare products that are appropriate for your skin type: Using skincare products that are formulated for your specific skin type can help to prevent and reverse signs of aging.

Incorporating anti-aging ingredients into your skincare routine: Ingredients such as retinoids, antioxidants, and hyaluronic acid can help to prevent and reverse signs of aging.

Using makeup techniques that accentuate natural beauty and minimize the appearance of aging: Techniques such as contouring, highlighting, and using natural-looking colors can help to create a more youthful and radiant appearance.

Consulting with a healthcare professional: Consulting with a healthcare professional can help you to understand your individual risk for age-related diseases and can help you to develop a personalized plan for maintaining overall health.

Experimenting with alternative treatments: Some alternative treatments such as acupuncture, hormone therapy, and anti-aging supplements may have potential benefits, but it is important to consult with a healthcare professional before starting any new treatment or therapy to ensure that it is safe and appropriate for you.

Be mindful of your genetics: Be mindful of your genetics and the risks that come with it, but also be aware of the fact that lifestyle choices and environmental factors

can have a big impact on your health
outcomes.

It is important to remember that aging is a
natural process and that there is no
one-size-fits-all solution for maintaining a
youthful, radiant appearance. Everyone's
skin and body is different, and what works
for one person may not work for another.
Therefore, it's important to find what
works best for you and to be consistent
with it.

9 798375 525167